# Let's Laugh At Men-o-Pause, It Can Help

Donna M. Workman

# DEDICATION

These poems are dedicated to my husband David Workman.

# CONTENTS

Donna M. Workman

Donna M. Workman

# ACKNOWLEDGMENTS

This book is dedicated to my husband DAVID WORKMAN. He reminded me when I first started my menopausal descent that I had said "Oh this will be easy and a piece of cake. No problem for me".

Was I a little naïve, I guess so as ten years later I am still experiencing crawly legs, suffering hot flashes, palpitations, and the cramps that goes along with it. How I manage to laugh at it is very much contributed to by him.

My husband has suffered also while it has been a part of both our lives. We all have to endure whatever comes our way. Yes, we women surely should get a very nice reward for our endurance; we also should give a reward to all our loved ones, who suffered from our ordeal.

So a special thank you to my nice husband David. I love you.

Also a special thank you to my editor, Lloyd Martin, who put many hours and thoughts, into making; Let's *Laugh at Menopause, It Can Help*, a reality. It has been a real joy working with him.
Still laughing and smiling.

Donna Mae.

Let's Laugh At Men-o-Pause

# Foreword

My sister called me the other day. After the initial greetings, she went on to say she must be pre-menopausal, because of certain physical and emotional developments in her life.

Upon hearing that I said "Oh not that you are going to have panic attacks". At that time I allowed a chuckle and thereupon, she stamped in my face that it was not a laughing matter.

Not a laughing matter indeed! Any man will tell you that a menopausal wife is like prickly cactus under your sheet. The sad thing with that situation is that she never wants to be like that. For all those who do not know, menopause is the "change of life" for a woman. This might sound coarse and unkind, but is a fact nonetheless; that an ugly caterpillar turns into a beautiful butterfly in a change of life, but a woman can metamorphosed into something foreign and ugly, at this juncture.

Therefore for a woman, in this case DONNA WORKMAN, to have been inspired to address this depressing subject in such a light, jocular and satirical way, has to be unique and unprecedented.

This should be read by every woman of a certain age, even husbands and anyone else who wishes women well and who wants to understand what they are going through, or will be going through.

This work has enabled me to appreciate how fortunate I am as a man who does not have to go through this change. Or is it really so? I am a bit scared, as she did say in one of her poems, that menopause is actually… *men on pause.*

I wish Donna all the best, and bestow all honor on her for stepping into this arena for the enlightenment and even entertainment of us all, on an otherwise, almost tabooed subject .

### LLOYD MARTIN.

Let's Laugh At Men-o-Pause

# WOMEN ONLY

You say up

And he says down

You say square

And he says round

So goes the night

When he is fast asleep

And you are all wound

What is all this men-o-pause about

You are cold

And I am hot

You say go

And I say STOP

Hey, I need help

And he says not

Is this the way it's going to be

Men-o-pause is not for men

It's just for me

1

## **WOMEN ONLY** (Cont'd)

For all the reason

Menopause is

For women only .

# A VERY LONG NIGHT

Say, go to sleep

...It's not for me

Can't you see

 It's almost three

There he lies

All fast asleep

I can only try, to count the sheep

Its men-o-pause

My friend and foe

It keeps me up and won't let go

I work so hard and wait for night

And then it bites

That is so not right

Oh men-o-pause

It is not so nice

I'd like to put it

On a block of ice.

# THE LEG SYNDROME

Here it comes

As sneaky as can be

...the itchy, scratchy, crawly sensation

To devour me

On my leg it starts

Then creeps to my heart

To make me sad

And frustrated

I tell you

Men-o-pause is

Underrated

Making me go berserk

Such a monster and a quirk

Menopause is not for me

I hate it and I am not pleased

And I wouldn't even

Give it to the dog

# THE LEG SYNDROME (Cont'd)

But give me a hammer

And I would smash it in pieces so fine

It would never again cross my mind.

# A NIGHT LIFE

Oh

If I could sleep

How happy I would be

Then I would know that menopause

Finally

Left me

To see that night

When it takes flight

Finally to be free

Of misery

But then I am too young

It surely got me on the run

Until when

When

When...

When I am

Too old.

# I AM HOT NOW

This is awful, as awful as can be

The temperature is on

And all on me

It's like a tea kettle about to lose its top

I feel so hot, hot –hot-hot

And I just can't stop

Men oh! Men-o-pause

Here it goes

The thermostat's broke

Give me the hose

I'd sprinkle the air

And let the water fly

...Just to cool down

And not to fry

So on it goes

The ups and downs

Today hot

# I AM HOT NOW (Cont'd)

Tomorrow not

It makes me frown

...Cant be my own

Men-0-pause

Please go away

So my normal heat

May come to stay.

# MENOPAUSAL MIGRAINE

Well, tell me

Have you ever had a migraine...

Because, I have too

What can you expect!

It's the menopause flu!!

It comes along just as quick as a bug

It bites and scratches and puts you under a rug

Oh the migraine

The lights need to be dimmed

When head feels like it wants to swim

I hate the migraine

The pain is sharp

And when it hurts

It's every part!

So go away migraine

And don't ever come back

You are not welcome

## MENOPAUSAL MIGRAINE (Cont'd)

For another attack

Go away and never come back

And that I say

Is that.

Donna M. Workman

# A QUICK HOT FLASH

I am getting hot now

The boiler is on

You can't imagine

This is so wrong

I feel like a fire

Pull the alarm

It is all so fast

My top just blew

I am all heated up

Right thru and thru

I need to have

This madness stop

No more hot flashes

No, no, not that

# A QUICK HOT FLASH (Cont'd)

...now I feel better

It's finally gone

But wait before I know it

It will be right back on

So hot flashes

Hot flashes one two three

What is it you really want with me

So take off the sweater

Even though its winter

Slim down the clothes

Bring me some water

Make them stop and come no more

Hot flashes, hot flashes...

Such a bore.

# HERE COMES THE NIGHT (SWEATS)

SO!

How can I sleep

And endure another night

When I feel my body

In such a terrible fright

You toss and turn

And if that's not the end

The night sweats start

Its unforgiving win

The sheets get wet

And I am sticking like glue too

I really feel like an unwanted Phee-u!!

The sleep is rare and the time is no fun

When I feel like slurp

In need of the sun

So go away night sweats

And all feelings of blue

# HERE COMES THE NIGHT (SWEATS) Cont'd

I can only say HELP!

And try to renew

The energy lost

The sweat I have drained

Will not even affect

My entire weight gained

I want my life back.

# ROLLER COASTER RIDE

IF YOU ARE A WOMAN

JUST BEYOND YOUR PRIME

LOOK OUT FOR MENOPAUSE

IT'S ABOUT TIME.

It comes upon you

And brings its ways

And soon your mind

Is rolling like uncontrollable waves

Menopause is really like a roller coaster ride

You just don't know about its side

You are up one minute

 And down the next

You think you are good then

Then comes the mix

Menopause is nasty and not kind

And kicks like a mule

On your behind

# ROLLER COASTER RIDE (Cont'd)

Oh yes

It makes you sad when you are not

Makes you feel down

When you are on top

So goes the time and its crazy effect!

Just ride it through

And don't eject.

# GOING THROUGH MEN-O-PAUSE

When you are going through

Men-o-pause

So many people tell you

What you should do

Here is a list-

Drink lots of water with lots of ice

Get lots of rest and don't stay up all night

Drink lots of tea and with honey is best

Keep your life calm and a lot less stress

Make carrot juice

And add an apple or two

Try to eat vegetables

And drink broth too

Read a good book and sip tea on the side

Make sure your grandkids

PLAY OUTSIDE!

...then there is the hubby who can only stand by

# GOING THROUGH MEN-O-PAUSE (Cont'd)

...and shake his head and watch you cry

OH!  MEN-OPAUSE, SO MANY EXPERTS TO HELP ME IT SEEMS!

Yet I cry on bending knees...

# TEN WAYS TO GO TO SLEEP ON A MEN-O-PAUSE NIGHT

Don't I wish they all would work!

For what it is worth!

One

The first step is to count from one to ten

If it doesn't work start over again

Two

Start counting those furry sheep

If one hundred goes by hopefully you'll sleep

Along comes the third

As donkeys fly by

You start count their tails and wonder why

The fourth is funny as funny can be

Now you're counting leaves on a tree

The fifth thing you do

Is massage your head

You think that might help to numb you instead

# TEN WAYS TO GO TO SLEEP ON A MEN-O-PAUSE NIGHT (Cont'd)

Six. Its getting late

You might consider the sleepy time tea

So late it will surely make you pee

Seven times seven you could try to count

Perhaps the clock's ticking can put you out

Eight. With blanket in hand

Up and down adjusting the fan

Nine. Position yourself again and again

And ten. Open your eyes

As it is now morning my friend.

# MEN-O-PAUSE AND EXERCISE

How many times

People say this to you

A father a mother a hubby or a friend

Do thirty minutes of walking

You'll feel better and even look trim

We all know it's true without a doubt

To walk and exercise is talked about

Yet so many excuses I can come up with

Because of this menopause I have to deal with

I am too tired too out of shape

I will go in a minute and won't be late

So the story goes and the days fly by

When exercise is what I truly deny

Maybe a partner a true blue friend

Can get me going and we'll fly like a wren

I need to exercise

# MEN-O-PAUSE AND EXERCISE (Cont'd)

This is true

Come with me

 We'll go as two

But then it got me

And I couldn't say why

I want to go

But only sit and cry.

# MEN-O-PAUSE

Do men go through men-o-pause

Many women would agree

That the men in men-o-pause

Is not just for me

We can see that men have their strange bouts

When they get older

Without a doubt!

Some have highs and some have lows

Could it be menopause

Do you suppose

I'd dare say without a doubt

They have the curse

We're talking about

When they get hot and we're still cold

Could it be left untold...

They may change and do some crazy things

Like wear goofy clothes and jingly rings

# MEN-O-PAUSE (Cont'd)

They may not act their age or even be nice

Have you ever seen it happen more than twice

Well we can guess and wonder

And so because

MEN-O-PAUSE

Is actually men on pause.

# ANXIETY AND MENOPAUSE

These two things

Can go hand in hand

So inseparable

Within that band

When you feel the pressure coming onto you

It makes it hard to work it through

Menopausal anxiety

That comes quickly your way

Can only make you hope

For a different day

Your mind is wild

And your heart beats quickly

And you feel that your life

Is on a slope that is slippery

Oh anxiety

And unfound fears

Can bring you down

# ANXIETY AND MENOPAUSE (Cont'd)

And your eyes, full of tears

My hands are sweaty

And my forehead perspires

When menopause comes

With uncanny desires

I can only imagine when

It is all through

I won't feel this way

And become unglued.

# WOMEN ON MENOPAUSE NEED FLOWERS TOO

Have you men ever thought this through

When your wife is down and menopausal too

There is one way you can help pick her up

Send her flowers and just shut up...

When you give her a flower

Let her know she's the rarest kind

Tell her you love her

And that she's on your mind

Send her a rose

A daisy is nice

Or perhaps a Jasmine

Would even suffice

...It isn't the best time

For a show

But the little thought

To let her know

# WOMEN ON MENOPAUSE NEED FLOWERS TOO(Cont'd)

That you really care

So remember

 Husband dear

At that time

To be really nice

Makes her feel

She's the spice of your life.

# OH NOT THAT(PANIC ATTACK)

When on menopause

It's a crazy time it seems

So many strange things happen

So many behind the scenes

One thing I've had and I hate to say

Is when panic attack has come my way

I don't know which way to go

Or how I can even think

The panic attack

Really does stink

I have fears that nearly knock me out

I really don't want to even go about

I'd rather stay home

And veg on the couch

It would be less stressful

See what its 'bout

I can only imagine

# OH NOT THAT (PANIC ATTACK) Cont'd

Better days lay ahead

When all is over

And no more this dread

So panic attacks are not for me

I long for the day

When

when I'm set free.

# MENOPAUSE EXERCISE

Take a deep breath

And put on your clogs

You're soon going

On a menopause log

Start the day off

With a gallon or two

Of good fresh water

And bottles with you

Take a long jog

And a real good hike

Before you know

You're out of sight

Remember not

The man waiting home

As on the face

This might bring a frown

Run a path that has been beaten down

# **MENOPAUSE EXERCISE** (Cont'd)

And let the sweat drip

As you circle around

When menopause hits

You're going through gears

But exercise can help

Get through those fears

Think good thoughts

And breathe deep from inside

And the tension soon will subside

So on you go

And get a good start

And hopefully, menopause

Will soon fall apart.

# A MENOPAUSAL DIARY

I thought about starting a diary

Of my menopausal journey

The thought came to me as I started to worry

The beginning starts with a bang

Then as it progressed

The intensities just all expand

I don't know how the end will ever come about

Because menopause is all my life's blowing out...

The diary will tell how days unfold

And of my dismay of really getting old

It may be a best seller

From the contents within

As I realized

To my chagrin

Oh my...oh my

Menopause's a sin

It had me frustrated and turning so that

# A MENOPAUSAL DIARY (Cont'd)

I know the story and can see the plot

In a diary I start and how long it will go

Not for me to really know

This for sure

It must come to end

When on this road

I turn the next bend.

Readers Notes